Common Reproductive Disorders in Cattle

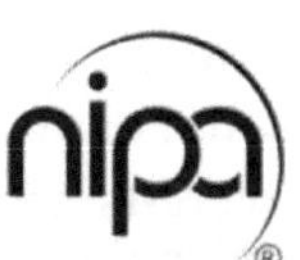

NIPA® GENX ELECTRONIC RESOURCES & SOLUTIONS P. LTD.
New Delhi-110 034

About the Author

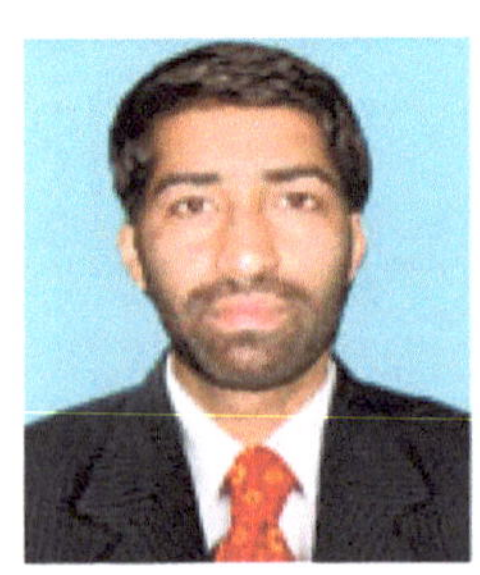

Dr. Khursheed Ahmad Sofi, is presently working as Assistant professor cum Junior Scientist (Senior Scale) in SKUAST- Kashmir, India. He did his M.V.Sc in Animal Reproduction, Gynaecology and Obstetrics as Junior Research Fellow (ICAR) from SKUAST-Kashmir and PhD in Veterinary Gynaecology and Obstetrics from CSKHPKV, Palampur-HP. He qualified ICAR NET in 2010, received Merit Scholarship and Certificate of Honour for PhD. He received Certificate of Appreciation as an Author (2018) from Veterinary Medicine-Open Journal and Certificate of Appreciation as an Editorial Board Member (2018 and 2020) from Veterinary Medicine-Open Journal. He is Life member (No. 1710) of Indian Society for the Study of Reproduction and Fertility (ISSRF) and The Indian Society for the Study of Animal Reproduction (ISSAR) (No. 3287). He has published 63 publications in both national and international reputed journals. Further, his research interests are in in vitro embryo production and cryopreservation especially vitrification of oocytes, ultrasonography and laparoscopy in animal reproduction and infertility.

Common Reproductive Disorders in Cattle Farmer's Guide

Khursheed Ahmad Sofi (PhD)
Assistant Professor, Senior Scale
Division of Veterinary Clinical Complex
Faculty of Veterinary Sciences and Animal Husbandry
Sher-e-Kashmir University of Agricultural Sciences and Technology-Kashmir
Srinagar- 190 006, Jammu and Kashmir, India

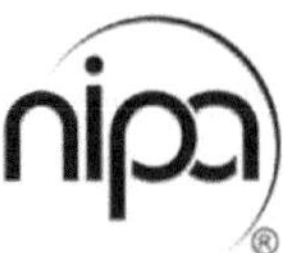

NIPA® GENX ELECTRONIC RESOURCES & SOLUTIONS P. LTD.
New Delhi-110 034

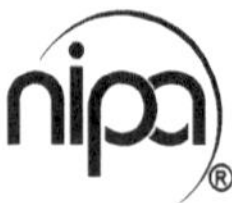

NIPA. GENX ELECTRONIC RESOURCES & SOLUTIONS P. LTD.

101,103, Vikas Surya Plaza, CU Block
L.S.C. Market, Pitam Pura, New Delhi-110 034
Ph : +91 11 27341616, 27341717, 27341718
E-mail: newindiapublishingagency@gmail.com
www: www.nipabooks.com

For customer assistance, please contact
Phone: + 91-11-27 34 17 17
Fax: + 91-11-27 34 16 16
E-Mail: feedbacks@nipabooks.com

Print ISBN: 9789-358-872-64-4

ebook ISBN: 978-93-58873-15-3

Composed and Designed by NIPA®.

Preface

I am pleased to offer this edition of "Common Reproductive Disorders in Cattle; Farmer's Guide" as an easy and comprehensible guide for dairy farmers. It covers many aspects of different reproductive diseases commonly found in dairy cattle related to infertility with practical information for farmers. Improving fertility is a common goal for dairy herds or livestock owners and getting cows pregnant in a timely manner is important in maintaining a profitable dairy business. Scientific management of dairy cattle is indispensable for achieving optimum reproductive efficiency and to reduce losses due to various reproductive diseases leading to infertility as infertility is one of the major causes for economic loss to farmers and making dairy farming economically unviable. Therefore, it is of utmost importance to manage the most probable causes leading to reproductive failures in cows with early intervention in order to reduce their economical impact in dairy cows and this can be possible through improving the knowhow of the farmers concerned with rearing of cattle as is expected with the help of this book.

We hope that the farmers especially will find this edition full of valuable and practical information and that this book will continue to have favorable influence on dairy cattle reproduction. Further, there is always scope for improvement and any suggestions or corrections if any may be communicated to the author.

Khursheed Ahmad Sofi

Contents

1

Repeat Breeding Syndrome in Cow

A cow is called repeat breeder when it has failed to conceive even after three or more number of services, has normal estrus cycle length, no abnormal vaginal discharge, no palpable abnormality in the reproductive tract, has calved at least once before and is less than ten years of age. Repeat breeding is one of the most important infertility problem faced by field veterinarians.

Causes

1) Fertilization failure
2) Early embryonic death

Main Points that Need to be Known by a Farmer About Repeat Breeding Cow

- Signs of estrus like vaginal discharge and its color, bellowing, mounting etc
- Time of estrus as observed by owner (morning, evening etc)
- Vaginal discharge whether clear or mucopurulent/purulent
- Duration of estrus
- Inter-estrous interval
- Number of inseminations
- Natural service or A.I
- A.I done by VAS / Non professional
- AI at dispensary or at Home
- Last calving date, whether normal or not (Dystocia, RFM, Metritis etc)
- Metestrous bleeding (MEB) present or not
- Deworming status and date
- Any treatment done

Management of Repeat Breeder Cow

- Check the animal for any reproductive problem by a qualified veterinarian and treat it.
- Provide the animal balanced ration with respect to minerals, vitamins which are essential for proper reproductive function.
- Provide the balanced ration so that the cow is not too fat or too lean.
- The body condition score at breeding time should be around 3.0 on 5 point scale.
- Regular deworming of cow with broad spectrum anthelmintic drug should be done.
- Observe the animal for estrus behavior at regular intervals on expected days.
- Bring the animal to the dispensary for A.I comfortably. Avoid any stress during this to and fro journey to animal as stress strongly reduces the chances of animal becoming pregnant.
- At estrus, inseminate the cow following A.M- P.M rule.
- Before A.I, rule out sub clinical endometritis (SCE) by White Side Test/Leucocyte Esterase test of cervico-vaginal mucus as sub clinical endometritis is the most common cause of failure of conception in repeat breeding cows. If found positive for SCE, skip A.I and administer broad spectrum antibiotic either intra-uterine or preferably parentally for 3 to 5 days followed by A.I on next heat.
- If estrus duration is more than 24 hrs, double A.I the cow at 12-24 hrs interval.
- Always ensure that the A.I has been done properly and scientifically. Ensure proper thawing and loading of A.I gun before insemination of cow.
- Always ensure that the A.I has been done cleanly and aseptically as any dirt or contamination at the time of A.I leads to not only failure of conception but also development of uterine infections like sub clinical endometritis, endometritis etc.
- Avoid use of any hormones at the time of A.I unless otherwise indicated by an expert.

- Progesterone @500mg (2ml) IM on Day 5 Post AI may be given for improvement of conception rate specifically in repeat breeding cows having history of metestral bleeding.
- GnRH Analogue @10 µg (2.5ml) IM on 12th Day Post AI may be given for improvement of conception rate specifically in repeat breeding cows having luteal insufficiency.

Who is to blame for Repeat breeding in cows????

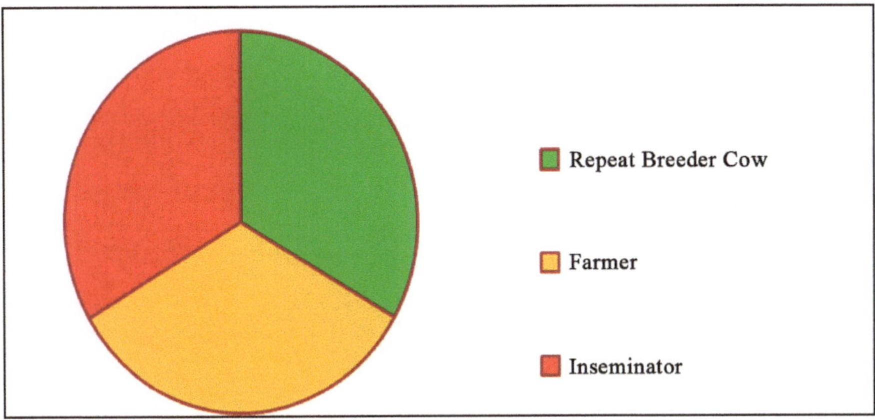

All are equally responsible

2

Anoestrum and its Management in Cow

Anoestrus in cows is a condition in which there is absence of observable estrus signs. Anoestrus in cattle is suspected when estrus in not expressed by the female animal or in case the farmer fails to detect it. Among reproductive problems, it is one of the most commonly occurring conditions in cattle. It affects the production and economics of a cow to a great extent and the economic losses occur due to increase in inter-calving interval, poor net calf crops, loss of production, expenses incurred on treatment etc. It is caused by multiple factors including mostly inadequate or unbalanced nutrition, environmental stress, uterine or ovarian pathologies and poor managemental practices.

Diagnosis

- Rectal examination of animal. The ovaries are small and smooth. Should be confirmed by repeated examinations at 10 days interval.
- Ultrasound examinations at regular intervals can be done to diagnose and confirm anestrous.
- Progesterone estimations at intervals of 10 days would aid in confirmation. Low progesterone levels at both times indicate true anestrous.

Management

In general, the management protocol for anoestrum cases involves the following steps:

• Improve Nutrition

- Feeding of concentrate mixture or grains, green fodder along with other roughages as per the requirements of an animal.

- **Supplement Vitamin and Minerals**
    - Standard vitamin and mineral mixtures at recommended doses (@30-50 gm daily orally) should be given especially during winter season.
- **Heat Inducers and fertility promoters**
    - Herbal heat inducers and fertility promoters like **Gestaforte bolus** etc. are very effective in anoestrum cases when given at recommended doses orally for 5-10 days.
- **Improve Managerial Practice**
    - Regular deworming to eradicate internal and external parasitism.
    - Proper housing and ventilation.
    - Elimination of stressful factors like heat, cold etc.
- **Specific Treatment**
    - GnRH analogues like **Buserelin Acetate injection** (20 µg or 5 ml, IM). May be repeated after 10 days.
    - Phosphorus injection @ 15 ml IM on 1st and 3rd day.
    - **Short term progestogens- CIDR, PRID or Ear implant** induces heat even in anestrous animals.
    - Progesterone injection followed by hCG or combination of progesterone + PMSG + estrogen.
    - Oestradiol Benzoate (2mg, IM) may be given in anoestrus condition in order to induce estrus.
    - Clomiphene citrate @ 300 mg daily for 5 days after drenching with $CuSO_4$ solution.

Point to remember

For economic consideration it is important to have heifers calve at least at 2.5 years of age and cows should give birth to calf after every 12-13 months.

3

Sub Estrus
Weak or Silent Estrus in Cow

Sub estrus (Weak or Silent Estrus) is a condition in which there are normal cyclical changes in the reproductive organs of a cow but the heat signs are not exhibited to a level of intensity as in normal cows leading to failure of estrus detection by a farmer. This condition is common during post partum period. It is a common reproductive problem in cattle affecting the productivity and economics of a cow due to increase in inter-calving interval, production loss, treatment expenses etc.

Causes

- Poor nutrition
- Seasonal stress
- Suckling
- Advanced age

Treatment

- Improving the managerial practice.
- Supplement Vitamin and Minerals: Give standard mineral mixtures at recommended doses orally.
- Heat Inducers: Herbal heat inducers like **Gestaforte** etc. are very effective when given at recommended doses orally for 5-10 days.
- Oestradiol Benzoate (2mg, IM) may be given in sub oestrus condition in order to enhance expression of estrus.
- Increased regular observation of animal for estrus signs. Provision of adequate lighting to improve estrus detection.
- Use of estrus detection aids.
- Use of teaser bulls

- Careful and frequent examination of cows, prediction and confirmation of estrus and breeding.
- Specific hormonal treatment and fixed time insemination - Highly effective.
- Unobserved estrum may be due to managerial deficiencies and short period of estrus.

4

Subclinical Endometritis in Cow

In subclinical endometritis (SCE), there is inflammation of the internal lining of uterus (endometrium). It is one of the major causes of repeat breeding in cattle and causes significant reduction of reproductive performance. Cervico-vaginal mucus in subclinical endometritis is clear in contrast to endometritis. It is also called cytological endometritis and is associated with increased proportion (percentage) of polymorphonuclear cells (PMN) in endometrial cytology samples. SCE affected cows have delayed first service and subsequent pregnancy causing significant economic losses due to reduction in reproductive performance, feed intake increase per lactation, milk yield reduction and increase in culling rate.

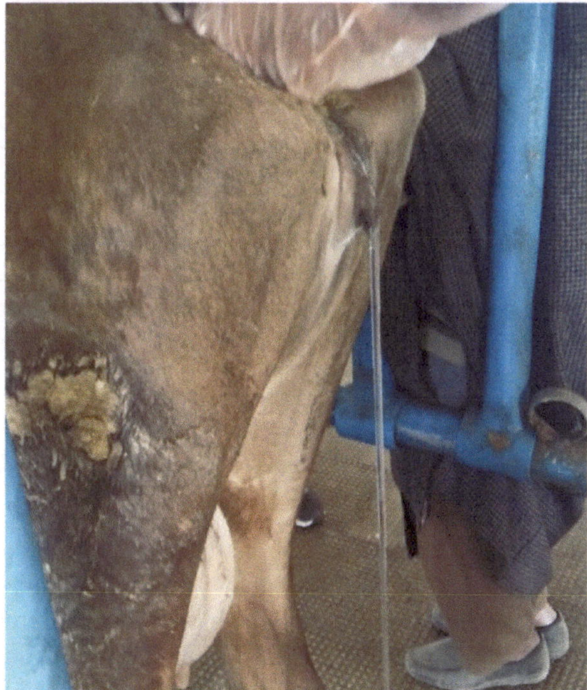

Clear vaginal mucous

Therapeutic Management

Subclinical endometritis is often self-limiting and the animal recovers from it after subsequent oestrous cycles. There are various intrauterine and systemic therapies that have been used for the management of subclinical endometritis in cattle and the commonly used therapies include

- **Lugol's Iodine:** In cows diagnosed with subclinical endometritis, solution of Lugol's iodine in diluted form in infused intra uterine for its treatment. Lugol's iodine infused intra uterine leads to endometrium irritation, stimulates uterine tone and enhances movement of neutrophils into uterine lumen. Lugol's iodine has advantages that it does not require a withdrawal period and does not pass into the milk except in the case of excess administration. Lugols Iodine may be given (0.3%, 30 ml Intra Uterine for 3 Days) as a cheap and safe therapeutic agent followed by AI on next estrus in subclinical endometritis affected cows.
- **Antibiotics:** Treatment of subclinical endometritis using antibiotics is targeted towards fertility improvement. Antibiotics that are to be used in subclinical endometritis affected cows should be effective against the main uterine pathogens and in the uterine environment. Currently, several treatment protocols for SCE are available in the literature i.e. Cephapirin, Ceftiofur, Levofloxacin-Ornidazole and α-Tocopherol combination, Levofloxacin etc. Levofloxacin given @ 4-5 mg/kg body wt. IM for 3 Days followed by AI on next estrus is also effective in subclinical endometritis affected cows.
- **Prostaglandins:** Prostaglandin F2α and its analogues have been used in subclinical endometritis for treatment due to their actions like CL luteolysis causing progesterone decrease with increase in estrogen concentration, ecbolic action and augmenting uterine PMN cells phagocytic activity.
- **Immuno-modulators:** In subclinical endometritis, different immune-modulators have been used like ***E. coli Lipopolysaccharide (E. coli LPS), Oyster glycogen, Proteolytic enzymes etc***
- **Herbal drugs:** Various herbal drugs containing herbal ingredients like *Aristolochia bactreata, Rubia cardifolia, Peganum harmala, Camiphora molmol* and *Lepadenia reticulata* stimulate uterine blood flow to uterus and are having ecbolic, anti-inflammatory and antibacterial actions thus, can be used as an alternative approach for subclinical endometritis treatment.

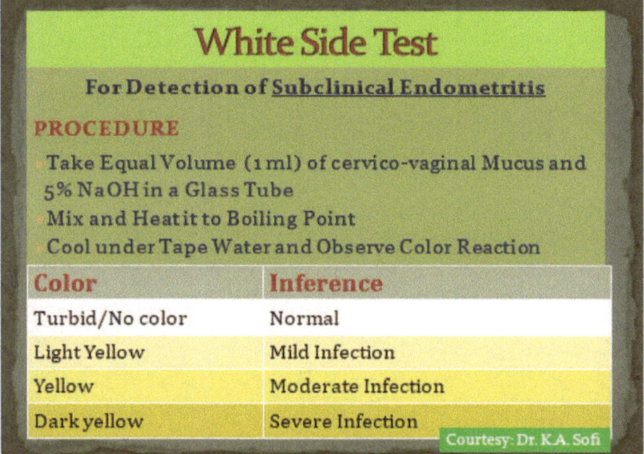

White Side Test for subclinical endometritis

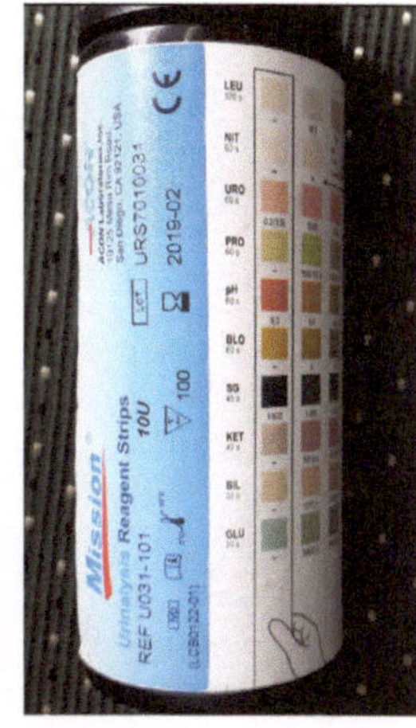

LE strips for diaganosis of Subclinical endometritis.

5

Endometritis in Cow

Endometritis in cow is actually the inflammation of endometrium that is inner lining of the uterus. It occurs after bacterial contamination of uterus at calving, during A.I. following dystocia, retention of placenta, abortion etc. There is expulsion of white or whitish-yellow muco-purulent discharge from vagina. The animal does not shows systemic signs like increase in temperature, increase in respiration rate, anorexia, toxemia etc as in metritis. However, the animal fails to conceive even after repeated inseminations.

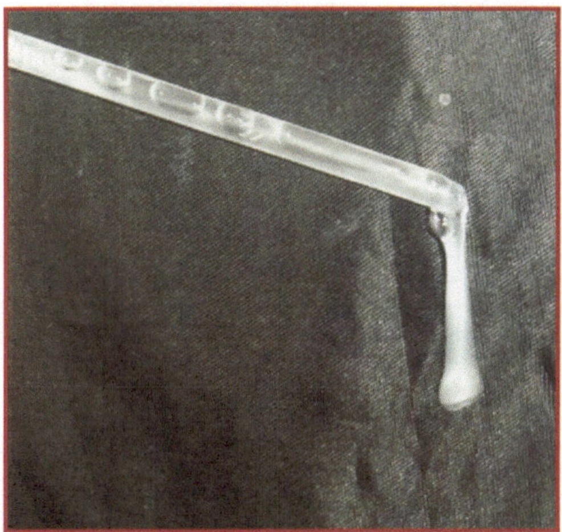

Whitish muco-purulent discharge

Clinical signs

- White or whitish-yellow muco-purulent vaginal discharge which comes out usually when a cow sits down.
- Copious muco-purulent discharge is observed at the time of estrus.
- There are no signs of systemic illness like in septic puerperal metritis.
- Repeat breeding and failure of conception are the most common symptoms of endometritis affected cattle.

Treatment

Therapeutic approach of endometritis includes:

- Antimicrobial therapy: Antimicrobial treatment may be done in endometritis affected cows either through intrauterine route or parental administration (Preferred) or even both. Currently, several treatment protocols for endometritis are available in the literature i.e. Cephapirin, Ceftiofur, Levofloxacin-Ornidazole and α-Tocopherol combination, Levofloxacin etc. Levofloxacin given @ 4-5 mg/kg body wt. IM for 3 Days is effective in endometritis affected cows.
- Hormonal therapy like oestradiol benzoate @ 2 mg (2 ml) IM, PGF2α analogue i.e. cloprostenol @ 500 μg (2ml) IM.
- Supportive therapy with oral herbal ecbolics like Uterivive, Uterotone, Uterifit etc., and oral calcium supplementation like Ascal Gold, Ostovet etc at recommended dosage.
- Vitamin B-complex with liver extract like Beekom-L (@10 ml/ animal) may be given intramuscular for 3-5 days.

6

Metritis in Cow

Metritis is a condition seen in cattle in which there is the inflammation of the entire thickness of uterine wall (endometrium, myometrium and serosa). When it occurs just after parturition, it is called puerperal metritis. It usually occurs after abnormal birth like in case of dystocia, abortion, RFM etc. The animal shows systemic signs like increase in temperature initially, increase in respiration rate, anorexia, toxemia etc. There is expulsion of large volume of foul smelling reddish to brown discharge from vagina frequently associated with straining. The expelled discharge from vagina is often with pieces of degenerating placenta.

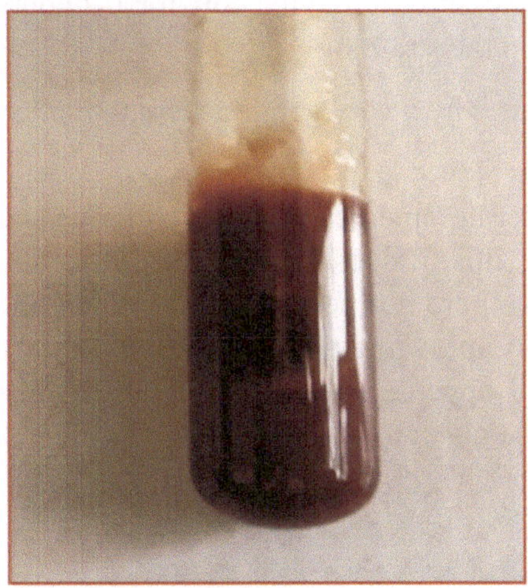

Reddish to brown discharge

Treatment

- Antimicrobial therapy e.g., Enrofloxacin, Levofloxacin, Ceftriazone, Ceftiofur etc. I/M or IV for several days until recovery occurs. Ceftiofur may be given in severe cases of metritis @ 1.1-2.2 mg/kg b.w. IM at 24 hours interval for 3-5 days. Levofloxacin may be given @ 4-5 mg/kg body wt. IM daily for 3-5 Days in metritis affected cows.

- Non steroidal anti-inflammatory drugs like Meloxicam @ 0.5 mg/kg b.w. at 24 hours interval.
- Antihistamines like Chlorpheniramine maleate, pheniramine maleate. Pheniramine maleate (Avilin-vet) may be given at the dose rate of 5-10 ml I/M.
- Glucocorticoid (Dexamethasone) should be used in severe case to prevent septic shock. Dose -10-30 mg (total dose) or 5 ml. I/M or I/V every 24 hours.
- Fluid and electrolytes: The intravenous infusion of large quantities of fluids and electrolytes is essential in the management of septic puerperal metritis. Large volume of isotonic fluids has been standard practice. Lactate Ringer's solution or a balanced electrolyte mixture should be given by IV infusion over several hours. Glucose should be included in the infusion fluids.
- Caudal epidural anesthesia using lignocaine 2% is used if the cow is straining repeatedly as it gives temporary relief to the cow for 1-2 hours and may cause cycle break and stop the straining.
- Remove the retained fetal membranes by a very gentle external traction otherwise leave it as such.
- Intrauterine medication: Intrauterine medication is controversial because in the acute puerperal metritis, it does not eliminate infection and all the layers of the uterine wall are not penetrated in intrauterine antibiotic therapy. After the initial improvement like when temperature approaches normal, resumption of appetite and cessation of diarrhea then, intrauterine antibiotics may be given to speed up recovery.
- Vitamin B-complex with liver extract may also be given to manage anorexia or decrease in appetite.
- Use of intravaginal probiotics as a new approach to prevent uterine infections.

Point to remember

Use of oestrogen is contraindicated in cases of acute puerperal metritis because oestrogens increase the contraction and blood flow in the uterus thereby increasing the absorption of bacterial toxins and thus, the case becomes more severe.

7

Retained Fetal Membranes (RFM) in Cow

Retained fetal membrane (RFM) in cow is a condition in which fetal membranes or placenta fail to separate and expelled by 12-24 hours after the birth of calf. It is a common in bovines and is usually associated with dystocia, abortion etc. Retained placenta in bovines predisposes the animal to uterine infection and thereby leads to infertility.

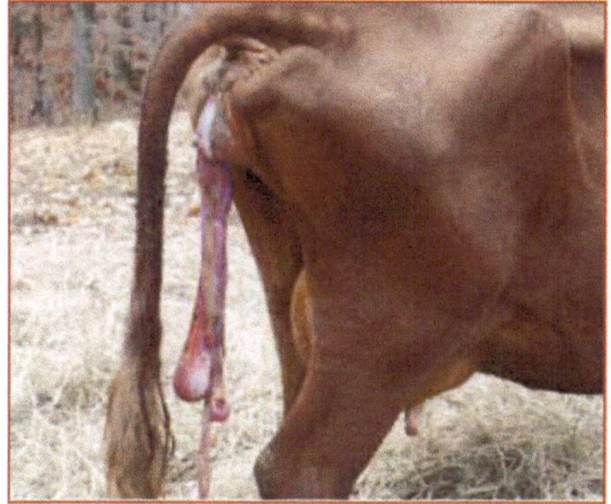

RFM in Cow

Clinical signs

Non infectious or low grade infection	Severe infection and/or prolonged duration
• Hanging of the placenta.	• Anorexia
• No foetid smell from the placenta.	• High fever and pulse rate
• Normal appetite, pulse and temperature.	• Reduced milk yield
• Milk yield normal.	• Straining
• Placenta is normal in colour, moist and glistening.	• Discolored and dry placenta with foetid smell

Treatment

Various treatment approaches have been used for animals with retained fetal membranes with controversial arguments. Treatment approaches that have been taken for management of retained fetal membranes in cows are as:

Administration of Ecbolic Agents

i. **Oxytocin:** 75-100 IU intramuscularly if used immediately after calving, reduces the rate of RFM.

ii. **Oestradiol Benzoate** (2mg, IM) may be given in RFM to aid in expulsion of placenta.

iii. **Indigenous preparations:** Many indigenous herbal preparations are available in the market for removal of retained placenta like Utrevive, Uterotone, Uterifit etc. These indigenous herbal preparations are used for the expulsion of retained placenta as well as to assist in manual removal of placenta. These herbal preparations are used with a loading dose on the first day followed by 100ml twice orally for 3-5 consecutive days. Calcium borogluconate may also be given to improve myometrium tone and to hasten expulsion of retained placenta.

Manual Removal

If normal expulsion of placenta fails even after the treatment with above mentioned drugs, then the placenta should be removed manually. However, cows should not be examined until 96 hours after calving as per the present recommendations and that the removal of placenta should be gentle and limited to the portion that gets spontaneously detached from the caruncles.

- Intrauterine treatment: After manual removal of placenta, intra uterine therapy should be done to prevent uterine infection. Many intrauterine preparations are available in the market like Lixen IU, Lenovo AP, Vodine IU, Metricef IU, C-flox-TZ *etc.* and these preparations are infused in the uterus for 3 to 5 days in suspension form.

- Parental antibiotics: If there is any chance of active infection, then parental antibiotics should be given for 3-5 days. Levofloxacin, Ceftiofur etc has a good effect.

- Antihistamines, non-steroidal anti-inflammatory drugs (NSAIDS) and liver extract should also be given.

- Use of intravaginal probiotics as a new approach to prevent uterine infections.

Point to remember

The manual removal of fetal membranes/ placenta in cows should not be attempted until 96 hours after calving and that removal after that period should be gentle and should be limited to the withdrawal of spontaneously detached placenta only.

8

Vaginal Prolapse in Cow

Vaginal prolapse in cow is a condition in which there is protrusion of whole or part of vagina including sometimes the part of cervix through the vulva. It occurs in cow mostly during last 2-3 months of gestation. It occurs due to excess secretion of estrogen from placenta, hypocalcaemia, inadequate exercise, bulky food like roughages etc. Sometimes occurs in non pregnant cows due to cystic ovaries, severe straining due to vaginal irritation etc.

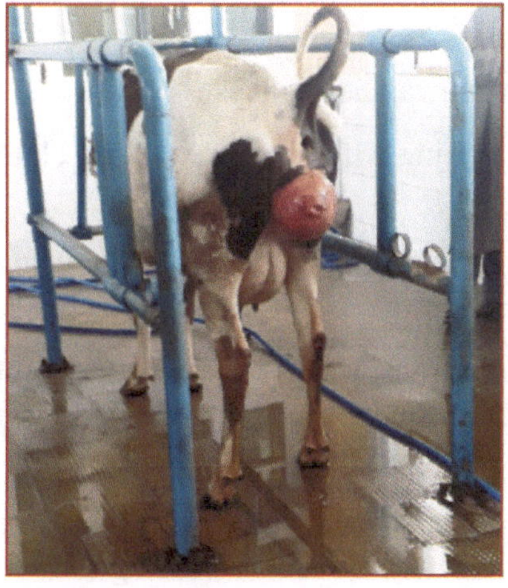

Cervo-Vaginal Prolapse

Main Predisposing Factors for Vaginal Prolapse

- Hypocalcaemia
- Inadequate exercise
- Bulky food
- Hormonal excesses and imbalances
- Excess dietary fiber
- Dietary estrogens and their precursors

- Sloping terrain
- Vaginal irritation due to injury or infection

Management

- Avoid the factors leading to vaginal prolapse like high estrogenic feed, inadequate exercise, bulky feeding at one time, hypocalcaemia, vaginal infection etc.
- In less severe cases (First degree prolapse), practice conservative methods like raising of rear quarters of animal, avoid bulky feeding at one time rather feeding in small quantity at frequent intervals, offer laxative feed to cow and progesterone may be given @ 500 mg (2ml) IM to counteract the effect of estrogen.
- Oral calcium supplementation like Ascal Gold, Ostovet etc at recommended dosage.
- Consult doctor as soon as possible when vaginal prolapse occurs.
- Keep the prolapsed part clean by wrapping with clean wet cotton cloth till the intervention is done.
- Take precautions to avoid rubbing of the prolapsed mass by a cow and keep the prolapsed mass safe from contamination with dirt, dung etc.
- In severe cases of prolapse (2nd and 3rd degree prolapse), proper treatment procedures (Reduction, Reposition and Retention) should be followed along with antibiotics, anti-inflammatory and antihistamine drugs.
- Local application of antibiotic cream and local anesthetic jelly like lignocain jelly should be applied twice daily to reduce straining etc
- Follow the treatment and advisory given by the expert properly.

9

Uterine Prolapse in Cow

Uterine prolapse also called casting of the **"Calf Bed"** in cow is a condition in which there is eversion of whole or part of uterus outside the vulva after its movement through dilated cervix and vagina. It occurs in cow after the birth of calf and mostly in dairy cows having given birth many times to a calf. It occurs due to hypocalcaemia, defective involution, inadequate exercise, excessive force applied during removal of calf etc.

Management

- Avoid factors leading to uterine prolapse especially hypocalcaemia, excessive force etc.
- Consult doctor as soon as possible when uterine prolapse occurs.
- Keep the prolapsed part clean by wrapping with clean wet cotton cloth till the intervention is done.
- Keep the prolapsed part above the ischial arch using clean wet cotton cloth till the intervention is done in order to prevent edema and hence facilitating easy repositioning.
- Take precautions to avoid rubbing of the prolapsed mass by a cow and keep the prolapsed mass safe from injury and contamination with dirt, dung etc..
- Consult doctor and ensure early repositioning of prolapsed uterus back to its normal anatomical position.
- Ensure complete replacement of the uterus.
- If retention sutures are applied.....
- Oxytocin should be given in order to restore uterine tone and speed up involution of uterus and thus to prevent recurrence of the prolapse.
- Calcium borogluconate therapy should be given even if the animal shows no clinical signs of hypocalcaemia together with parental antibiotics.
- Follow the treatment and advisory properly.

Point to remember

Always check the animal for any recurrence and presence of any part of uterine prolapse in the vaginal canal by 24 hrs after retention sutures like Buhner's suture applied to the animal.

10

Pyometra in Cow

Pyometra meaning "pus filled uterus" is a condition in cow which is characterized by progressive accumulation of pus in the uterus, presence of persisting CL, absence of estrus and regular estrus cycles and a closed cervix. Pyometra occurs following chronic endometritis in most cases as uterus fails to produce endogenous CL regressing agent i.e. PGF2α. So, the CL of diestrus persists resulting in failure of elimination of uterine infection as the animal remains under the continuous influence of progesterone. Progesterone production from the persistent CL causes closure of cervix, pus accumulation in the uterus and consequently leading to enlargement and distension of uterus. Pyometra usually results after insemination following contamination of the uterus at the time of insemination and venereal infection causing embryonic death such as Trichomonas fetus. Death of the fetus and invasion of the uterus by organisms like A. pyogenes also cause pyometra. F. necrophorum and T. pyogenes are the common pathogenic bacteria found in purulent material of cows with pyometra. Diagnosis can be easily and accurately done by ultrasonography.

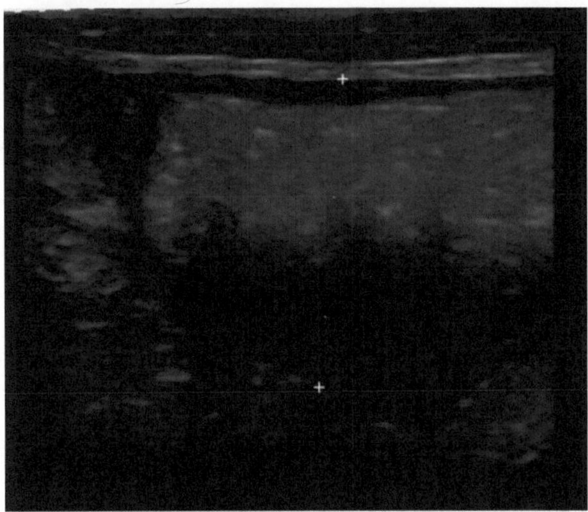

USG image of Pus filled Uterus

Symptoms and Diagnosis

Cows with pyometra show few or no signs of ill health but there is absence of cyclical activity and presence of an intermittent vaginal discharge when the cow lies down, urinates or defecates. The uterine horns are enlarged and distended as the cervix remains closed and the purulent material accumulates within the uterine lumen. Diagnosis of pyometra is done based on history and per rectal examination. However, diagnosis of pyometra in cattle can be easily and accurately done by trans rectal ultrasonography.

Management

- The treatment of choice in pyometra cases is PGF2α or its analogues like cloprostenol @ 500 μg (2ml) IM. PGF2α or its analogues cause corpus luteum regression, cervix dilatation, expulsion of the uterine purulent material and resumption of estrus and estrus cyclicity.
- Antimicrobial therapy either parental (Preferable) or intrauterine or both: Currently, several treatment protocols are available in the literature i.e. use of Cephapirin, Ceftiofur, Levofloxacin-Ornidazole and α-Tocopherol combination, Levofloxacin etc (for 3-5 days). Ceftiofur may be given @ 1.1-2.2 mg/kg b.w. IM at 24 hours interval for 3-5 days. Levofloxacin may be given @ 4-5 mg/kg body wt. IM daily for 3-5 Days in pyometra affected cows.
- Supportive therapy with oral herbal ecbolics, calcium supplementation etc
- Vitamin B-complex with liver extract should be given.
- Improving the managerial practice and to avoid infection of the reproductive tract at the time of A.I etc.
- Use of intravaginal probiotics has also been reported as a new approach to prevent uterine infections.

11

Uterine Torsion in Cow

Uterine torsion in cow is actually the rotation of the pregnant uterus on its longitudinal axis and usually occurs before onset or during late first stage of parturition but rarely encountered during early second stage of parturition. In cattle, uterine torsion involves both gravid and non gravid horns because of strong intercornual ligament and distension of uterine horn and body with placenta and fluid. The remarkable feature of uterine torsion is its association with advanced pregnancy and process of parturition in cow.

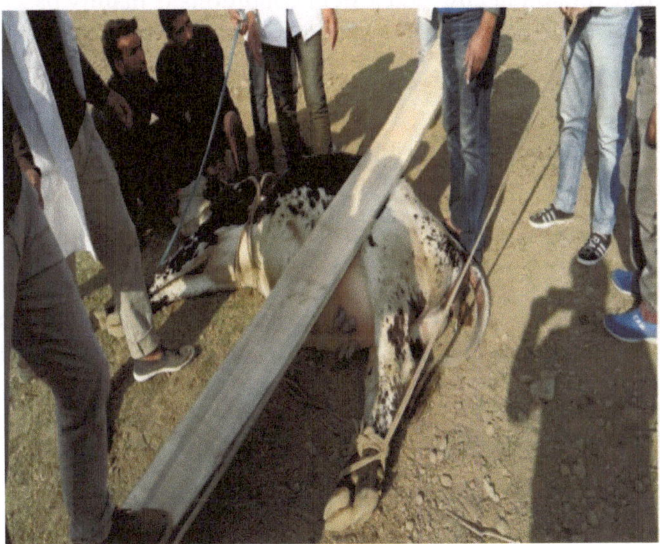

Detorsion in cow

Symptoms

The symptoms shown by cow having uterine torsion depends upon the degree of torsion with no symptoms in 45-90° or even 180° torsion. However, torsion of 180° or more is associated with following symptoms as:

• Anorexia • Constipation • Lack of rumination • Weak and slow rumen contractions	• Rapid pulse rate • Restlessness or colicy signs • Treading and tail switching

Symptoms may be confused with traumatic gastritis, indigestion, pyelonephritis or intestinal intussusception

In sever cases of uterine torsion, the symtoms include

• Complete anorexia and Constipation • Complete lack of rumination and rumen activity • Fetid diarhoea • Very rapid and weak pulse	• Rapid respiration and expiratory grunt • Normal to subnormal body temperature • Cold extremities • Shock collapse and death may occur within 24-72 hrs.

Diagnosis of Uterine Torsion in Cow

The daignosis of uterine torsion in cow under field conditions is mainly based of history, pervaginal examination and per rectal examination

History

- Symptoms like anorexia and Constipation, Lack of rumination and rumen activity, indigestion etc
- Prolonged first stage of parturition in uterine torsion causing dystocia
- Abdominal straining characteristics of second stage of labour is either absent or mild because twisted birth canal prevents entrance of fetus into pelvis- necessary prerequisite for initiation of normal abdominal straining.

Per Vaginal Examination

- If hand is inserted into vagina, it cannot be passed easily towards cervix.
- Twisting of hand indicates whether torsion is clockwise (Right) or anti-clockwise (Left).
- Starting from dorsum of vagina,
  - If the folds spiral forward and downward to the left or counterclockwise- Left torsion is present
  - If the folds spiral forward and downward to the right or clockwise- Right torsion is present

- Dorsal commissure of vulva is pulled forward and left in case of left torsion and forward and right in case of right torsion.
- Intensity of twisting or stenosis of birth canal indicates severity of torsion.
- Birth-canal is narrow and stenosed in region of anterior vagina,
- If torsion is greater than 180°-It is usually impossible to pass hand through twisted portion of birth canal.
- If torsion is less than 180°, the obstetrician's hand may be passed through birth canal to palpate the foetus.

Per Rectal Examination

- Where the site of twist is precervical, the vagina is much less involved and diagnosis is assisted by palpating the uterus per rectum.
- On rectal examination, twisted uterine horn can be felt and broad ligament on the side of torsion is rotated downwards sometime palpable under the uterus and ligament on opposite side is tense and stretched and crossing to the opposite side.
- Positive diagnosis of uterine torsion should thus, be based on location of broad ligaments palpated per rectum.
- Position of fetus indicate degree of torsion
- Dorso-pubic position of fetus occurs when the torsion is 180°

Management of Uterine Torsion in Cow

Uterine torsion in cow under field conditions is managed by Rolling of dam, Schaffer's method and lastly by caesarean section.

Rolling of Dam

- Ascertain the side of torsion.
- Cast the animal in lateral recumbency on the same side as the direction of torsion.
- The front and hind limbs are secured separately.
- Keep hand in birth canal and grasp the foetal part (if cervix is dilated).
- Roll the cow in the same direction of torsion.

- After cow has been rolled through 180°, her body must be pushed slowly over legs and sternum to bring back the same position to continue rolling in the same direction.
- Examine the vaginal passage to find out whether rolling is effective or not. If the rolling is effective, the spiral folds and stenosis of birth canal starts to disappear. If the rolling is in wrong direction, vaginal folds become more tight.
- After each two or three rapid rotations of the cow's body, the birth-canal should be examined.
- Occasionally, there may be a rush of foetal fluids from the uterus as the torsion is relieved.
- After correction of torsion, the foetus should be pulled out by applying forced traction as soon as possible.

Schaffer's Method

- It is a modification of rolling method.
- Cow is casted on the same side as direction of torsion. Legs are tied in the same manner as in the above method.
- A plank **9 to 12 feet long** and **8 to 12 inches wide** is placed over abdomen while other end of plank should be on the ground.
- An assistant stands on lower end of plank and cow is slowly rolled in the same direction of torsion.
- Determine by placing hand in the birth canal, whether torsion is being relieved or not.

Prognosis

Prognosis of uterine torsion in cow depends on degree of torsion, severity of symptoms and duration of torsion.

Good	Poor
• Mild cases without symptoms	• Advanced, severe and neglected cases
• 90° or less usually, occasionally 180°	• Fetus is usually dead
• 180 to 270° causing definite symptoms but diagnosed and treated early	• Prognosis is poor for life and fertility of dam

12

Cystic Ovarian Disease in Cattle

Cystic ovarian disease (Cystic ovarian degenertaion or ovarian cysts) is a common ovarian dysfunction in cattle and causes huge economic loss to farmers due to its high incidence and negative impact on the reproductive performance of cow. Animals having cysts on ovary result in anoestrum as the most significant clinical sign. Althouugh the exact cause that leads to cystic ovarian disease is not yet fully clear but altered release of LH hormone is the most accepted hypothesis.

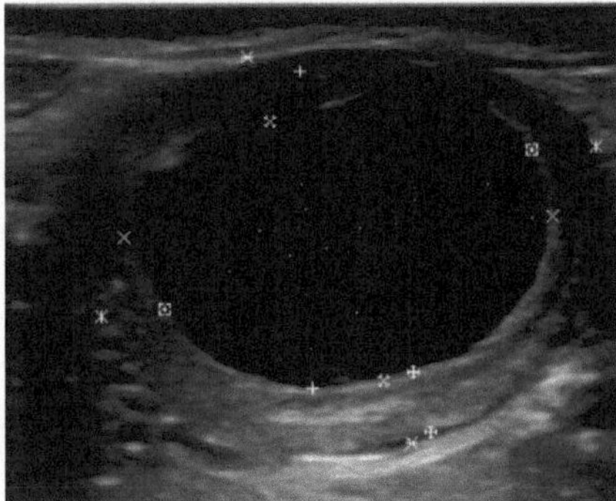

Luteal cyst on ovary (USG)

Cystic ovarian disease in usually defined as

- One or more fluid filled structures ≥2.5 cm diameter present on ovary
- Persistenting for 10 days or longer
- Aberrant reproductive function

The more recent definition describes this ovarian cystic condition as follicular like structures of at least 17 mm in diameter that persist on the ovary without CL for more than 6 days and clearly interfering with normal cyclicity.

Follicular Cyst	Luteal Cyst
• Soft, thin walled ≥ 2.5 cm diameter • Frequently multiple in one or both ovaries • Thickness of cyst wall <3mm • Low peripheral blood P4 levels • Anoestrus or nymphomaniacal	• Thick walled ≥ 2.5 cm diameter • Thickness of cyst wall >3mm • High peripheral blood P4 levels • Anoestrus

Main Predisposing Causes

• Hereditary • High milk yield • Season	• Stress • Negative energy balance • Age

Diagnosis

- **Per rectal examination, Ultrasonography**

Clinical Signs

• Nymphomania • Frequent and copious discharge of clear mucous • Relaxation of sacrosciatic and sacroiliac ligaments • Aggressive sexual behaviour	• Erratic milk production • Irregular interoestrous interval • Anoestrus: key clinical sign • Development of musculine physical traits

Management

- Avoid the factors predisposing to cystic ovarian disease like negative energy balance, stress etc.
- Hormonal treatment like hCG (3000 IU), GnRH (20 µg) etc
- Specifict teatment like GnRH analogue (Busereline acetate @ 20 µg IM) for treating folllicular cysts and PGF2α (Cloprostenol @ 500 µg IM) for treating luteal cysts.
- GnRH plus PGF2α plus GnRH (Ovsynch) protocol: best treatment especially under field conditions when specific treatment for follicular or luteal cyst is not feasible due to lack of accuarcy of diagnosing the typeof cyst present.
- Progesterone withdrawal treatment like intravaginal progesterone implants for 9-12 days.

13

Estrus in Cow

Estrus is referred to as the period of estrous cycle during which the female animal allows the male for mating. It is the period of estrous cycle during which insemination is done to female animal so that the animal will become pregnant. During estrus, cow usually seeks out the male and 'stands' for him to mate her. In all domestic species, Ovulation occurs during this phase of the cycle but in case of cow, ovulation occurs about 12 hours after the end of estrus period.

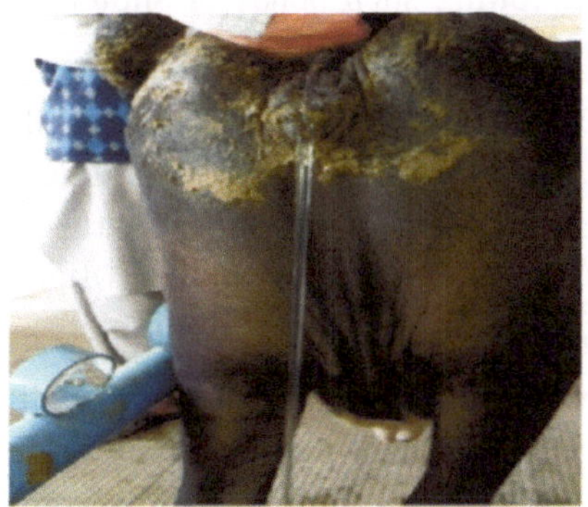

Hanging cervico vaginal mucous

Estrus Signs

It is essential to understand the primary and secondary signs of heat in order to achieve accurate and efficient heat detection; so that A.I is done at appropriate time and maximum chances are there that the cow will get pregnant after A.I.

a) Primary Sign

A cow standing to be mounted is the most accurate sign of estrus. *Standing heat* is the most sexually intensive period of the estrous cycle during which the cow stands still and allows mounting by other cows or bull or move forward slightly due to weight of the mounting animal. However, Cows that are not in true estrus move away quickly when mounting is attempted by other cows or bull. The average duration of standing heat in cow is 15 to 18 hours, although it may vary from 8 to 30 hours among cows. A cow in estrous usually stands to be mounted 20 to 55 times during her estrous period. In order for standing behavior to be expressed, cattle obviously must be allowed to interact. The expression of heat is due to the elevated level of estrogen in the blood when progesterone is very low. Occasionally cows in early pregnancy, approaching the end of pregnancy, or with ovarian follicular cysts have similar hormonal relationships and may express signs of heat.

b) Secondary Signs

Secondary signs vary in duration and intensity. These signs may occur before, during, or after standing heat and the farmer should use these signs as clues or watch the specific cow more closely for standing behavior.

i. **Mounting other cows:** Cattle that exhibit this behavior may be in heat or approaching towards estrus. Although mounting cannot be used as a true primary sign of heat, cows exhibiting such behavior should be observed closely for standing behavior.

ii. **Mucus discharge:** Long viscous, clear elastic strands of mucus generally hang from the vulva as an indirect result of elevated estrogen levels. Sometimes, however, the mucus does not appear externally until the cow is palpated during insemination and the mucus is expelled. Mucus also may be smeared on the tail, thighs, flanks, or perineal region.

iii. **Swelling and reddening of the vulva:** During estrus, the vulva swells and becomes moist, congested and red but remains pale when animal is not in heat.

iv. **Bellowing, restlessness, and trailing:** Cows in heat are more restless and alert to their surroundings and bellow more frequently during estrus. Although these are not definitive signs of heat, cows exhibiting such behavior should be kept under constant observation for standing behavior and other estrus signs.

v. **Rubbed tail head hair and dirty flanks:** In free ranging animals the hair on the tail head is rubbed, legs and flanks may be smeared with mud or manure as a consequence of being mounted by male.

vi. **Chin resting and back rubbing:**

vii. **Sniffing genitalia:** Sniffing the genitalia and licking the vulva of other cows occur much more frequently with cows in pro-estrus and estrus.

viii. **Head raising and lip curling:** Generally this activity follows sniffing of the genitalia and occurs more frequently if the cow being investigated is in heat and urinates.

ix. **Decreased feed intake and milk yield:** Estrous cows spend less time feeding. Some studies also have reported decreased milk yield during estrus.

Metestrous Bleeding

Some cows and most heifers have a bloody mucus discharge one to three days after estrus called metestrous bleeding. Presence of such bloody mucus discharge indirectly indicates that the cow was in heat and does not mean that she failed to conceive. However, such animals need to be observed carefully for a return to heat in 18 or 19 days if A.I has not been done at the estrus observed before this metestrous bleeding. However, repeat breeding cows having history of metestrous bleeding may be given hormonal therapy after A.I as metestrous bleeding has been seen associated with luteal insufficiency and hence leading to failure of conception in such cows.

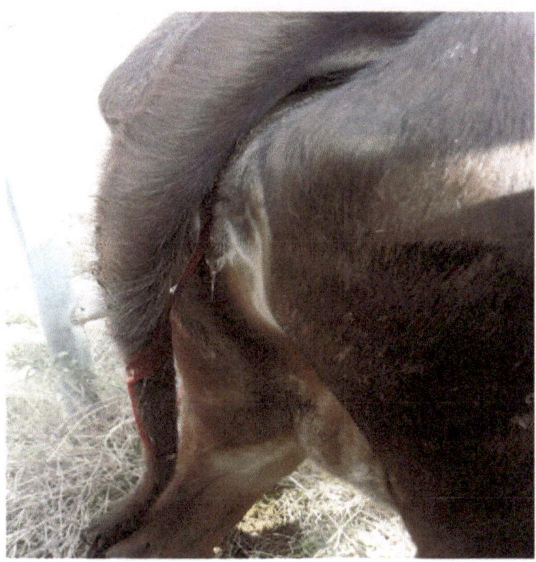

Metestral bleeding in cow

14

Artificial Insemination in Cow

Artificial insemination (AI) is a technique in which sperm cells loaded in straws and stored in liquid nitrogen are thawed and manually deposited into the reproductive tract of a female animal at estrus. The recto-vaginal technique is the most commonly used method for artificial insemination in cattle. In order to increase the probability of pregnancy, the animal in estrus should be inseminated at proper time not too early or late. To achieve highest fertility, a cow first observed in estrus in the morning should be bred late in the afternoon that same day. Similarly, a cow first observed in estrus in the evening should be bred the following morning. This AM-PM system is easy to follow and under most conditions result in good conception rate. Compared to natural service, artificial insemination is desired as it helps in preventing spread of venereal diseases and therefore reduces incidence of infertility.

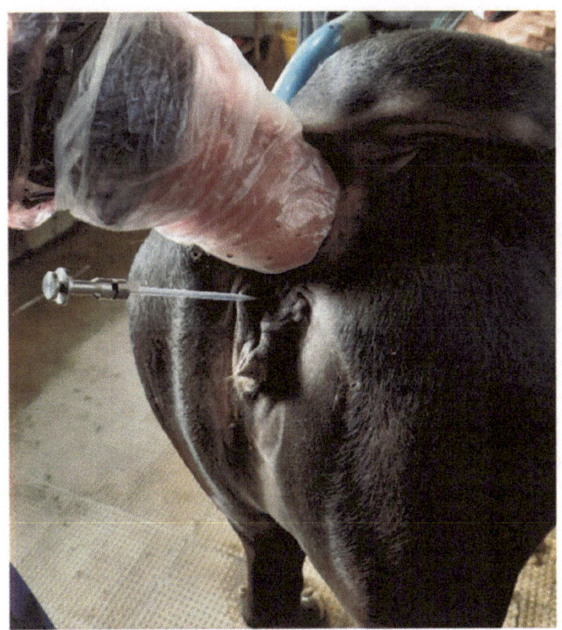

Main factors that influence the conception rate following artificial insemination in cattle are

- Proper estrous detection followed by artificial insemination at optimum stage of estrus not too early or too late but towards the end of estrus.
- The cow should be in optimum body condition score at the time of insemination.
- Proper storage and handling of frozen semen that is used for artificial insemination.
- Proper thawing and loading of frozen semen straws used for artificial insemination.
- Avoid cold shock to semen after thawing and loading of frozen semen straws in insemination gun.
- Correct insemination technique and proper deposition of semen at recommended site as per scientific guidelines.
- Maintenance of all aseptic measures to ensure contamination free artificial insemination.
- Avoid all factors leading to stress before and after artificial insemination.

Artificial Insemination Technique in Cattle

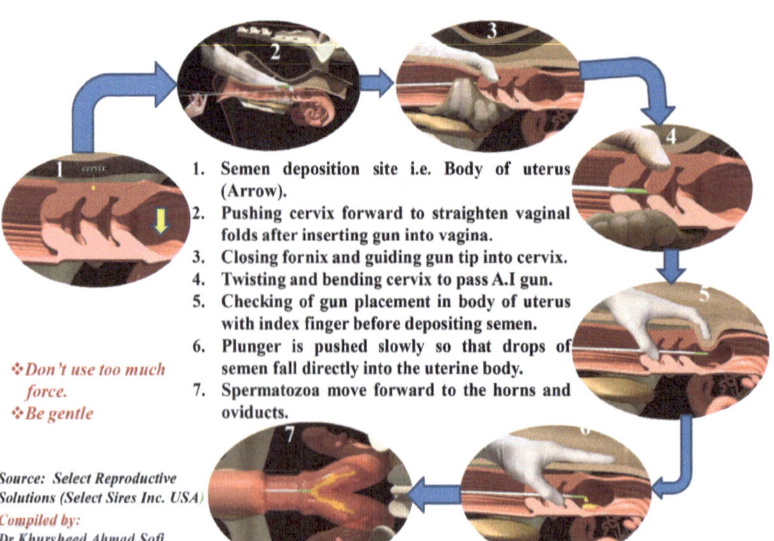

15

Pregnancy Diagnosis in Cow

The diagnosis of pregnancy (Cyesiognosis) was desired earlier by farmers for curiosity, but currently early pregnancy diagnosis is considered essential for economically viable and profitable dairy farming. Clinical methods are commonly used for pregnancy diagnosis in cattle with recto genital palpation and trans-rectal ultrasonography as the methods of choice for an accurate and early pregnancy diagnosis.

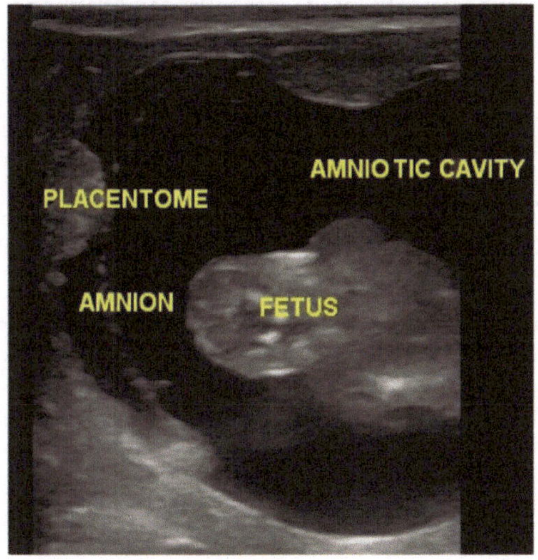

Visual Methods

These are important for a farmer although the accuracy is not comparable to other used methods like recto genital palpation but these visual observations give an important cue to farmer about the pregnancy status of cow. Some of importance for a farmer as follows

i) **Non return to estrus:** Not return to estrus after around 21 days of mating or A.I gives an indication that the animal may be pregnant. However, there are reasons other than pregnancy due to which the animal may not return to estrus and is also non pregnant.

ii) **Increase in the size of abdomen:** In advanced pregnancy, there is increase in size of abdomen.

iii) **Development of udder:** It is important as an indication of pregnancy especially in dairy heifers (4 months onwards) but in multiparous animals, it is often not evident until the final 1 to 4 weeks of pregnancy.

iv) **Movements of fetus:** Movements of fetus is visible externally on the right side in cows around 6 months onwards of gestation.

Recto-Genital Palpation

Trans-rectal palpation is the oldest and extensively used clinical method for diagnosis of pregnancy in cattle. Recto-genital palpation (with some limitations) in large domestic animal like cattle is the easiest, cheapest and fastest method of pregnancy diagnosis. There is no harm to the animal and its fetus in recto-genital palpation, when performed carefully for pregnancy diagnosis and can give accurate diagnosis of pregnancy after day 35 of mating or A.I.in cattle.

Ultrasonography

Using trans rectal ultrasonography, pregnancy can be accurately diagnosed in cattle around day **28-30** of mating or A.I. using a trans-rectal linear array probe of 5.0 to 7.5 MHz.

Point to remember

It is always advisable to have the cow checked for pregnancy diagnosis at least by 2 months after A.I/Natural service if the cow has not been observed in estrus after last breeding.

16

Prophylactic Vaccination for Cattle

Vaccination of cattle and prevention of diseases causing huge economic losses is very much essential for economic rearing of livestock as prophylactic and strategic vaccination helps in development of immunity against the vaccinated diseases thereby prevents the animals from developing such infections and consequent diseases. Animals should be vaccinated at specific age and at definite time intervals for optimal protection against the diseases.

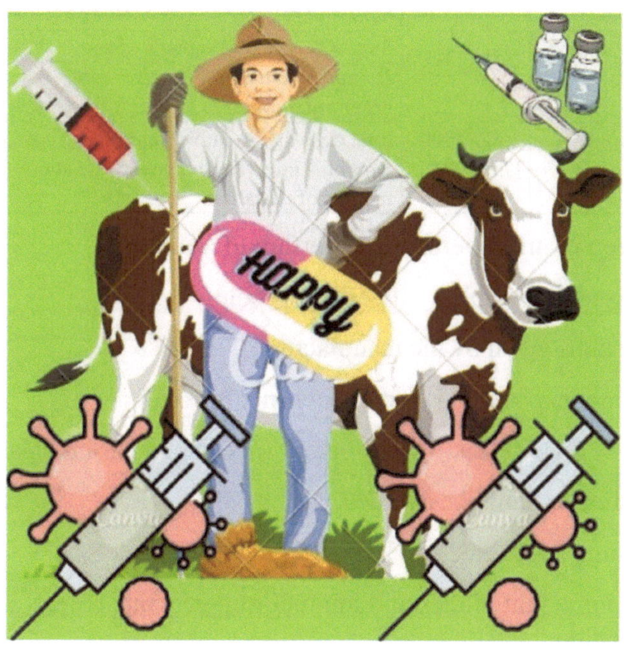

Vaccination Schedule

(Source: https://kvk.icar.gov.in/API/Content/PPupload/k0347_10.pdf)

Disease	Vaccine	Dose & Route	Schedule
FMD	FMD inactivated polyvalent vaccine	2ml, IM	First dose at 4 months of age, Booster at 6 months and then Repeat at every 6 months interval.
Hemorrhagic septicemia	H.S oil adjuvant vaccine	2ml, IM or S/C	First dose at 4-6 months of age and then Repeat every year preferably before rainy season (May-June).
Anthrax	Anthrax live spore vaccine	1ml, IM	First dose at 6 months of age and then Repeat at every year preferably in the month of May to June.
Black Quarter	Polyvalent (A, B, Q) vaccine	2-3ml, S/C	First Dose at 6 months of age and then Repeat every year, preferably before monsoon season.
Brucellosis	Brucella abortus Strain -19 live vaccine	2ml, S/C	Single Dose at 4-8 months of age ***Do not vaccinate male calves and pregnant animals***
Tetanus	Tetanus toxoid vaccine	1500-3000 Units, IM	First dose at 1 month of age, Booster at 6 months interval. Pregnant cattle at 6-7 months of gestation.

Important points to keep in mind before vaccination of animals

- Always use sterilized disposable syringes and needle.
- Follow the instructions given by the manufacturer.
- Ensure vaccine is not expired and cold chain is not broken.
- Deworming must be done at least 1 week before vaccinating the animals.
- Sick and weak animals should be avoided
- Avoid stress to animals at least 2 weeks post vaccination.
- Avoid administration of antibiotics and immune-suppressants at least 2 weeks post vaccination

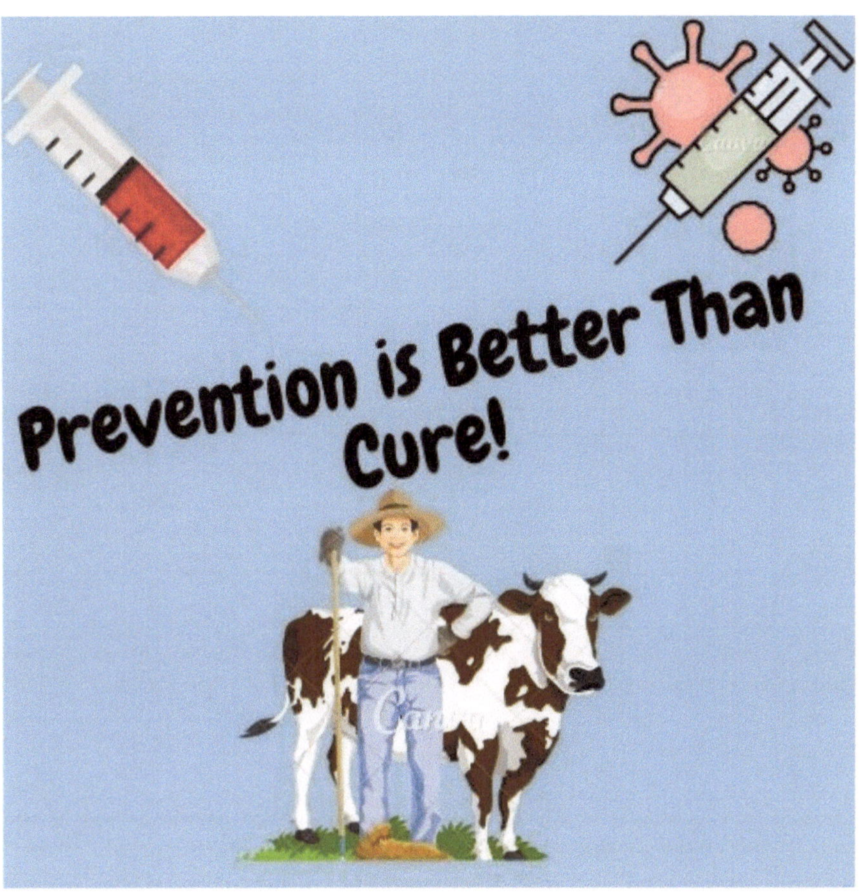
Prevention is Better Than
Cure!

17

Deworming Schedule for Cattle

Regular deworming of cattle including young stock is essential for economic rearing as sever parasitic infection leads to reduced feed intake, decreased reproductive performance, lower milk production, decreased growth rate and increased incidence of diseases. So, deworming as per scientific schedule and dose rate is a must for animals to keep away these profit eating parasites.

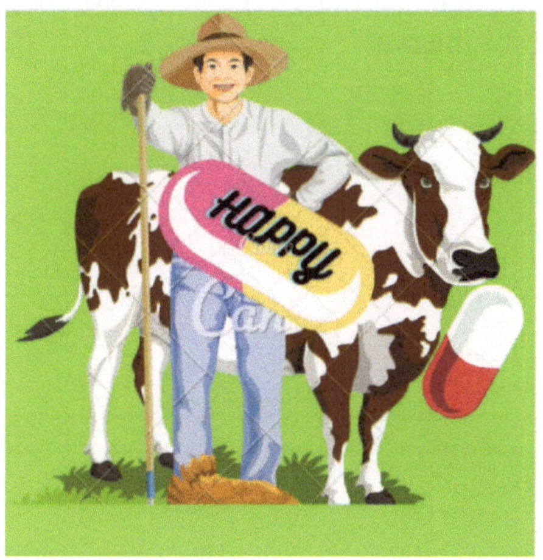

Calves

- From first week onwards of birth of calf, deworming should be started.
- For first 6 months of birth of calf, deworming should be done every month and thereafter once in 3 months.
- Deworming drugs that are to be used along with the dose and regimen need to be properly followed after consulting the professional veterinary doctor.
- It is very important to avoid over dosing and under dosing of deworming drugs in order to reduce the side effects and drug resistance.

Control measures

- Regular prophylactic deworming of animals using potent anthelmintic.
- Deworming drug should be preferably changed at frequent intervals in order to avoid resistance in animals.
- Therapeutic deworming of animals should be made based on fecal examination and egg count.
- Maintenance of good hygiene and sanitation of animal houses and feeders is important to control parasitic load.
- Vector and intermediate host control is also very essential for control of parasitic infection in animals.
- Adult animals under normal conditions should be given deworming drug at least twice a year at 6 months interval.

18

Care of Newborn Calf

Calves play an important role in the dairy development and successful growth of young calves to mature stage is required for herd replacement and to get economic returns when they are sold. Good calf-care is important for sustenance of the dairy form and preservation and maintenance of good quality germplasm.

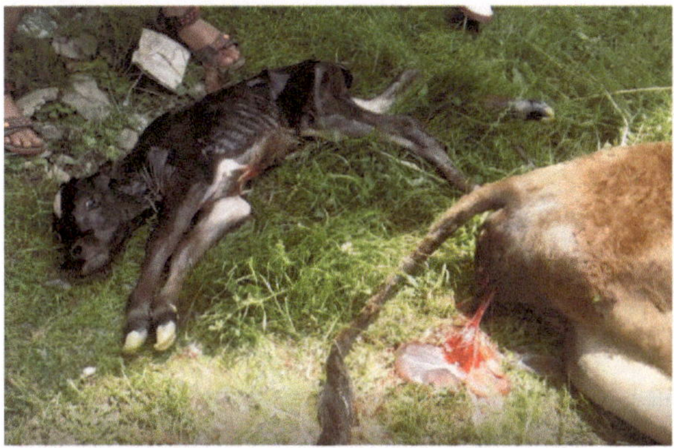

The most critical period of a calf's life is the first hour after birth, termed the **"Golden Hour"**. Correct calf management and feeding practices during this time influence the ensuing health and development throughout its life, and its overall lifetime performance. An assessment of the calf's vigour should be made immediately after calving. The following individual indicators should be monitored: external stimuli responsiveness, muscle tone, sucking reflex, the time calf takes to lift its head and the first standing. Normal time frames for some indicators of calf vigour are

- *Newborn calf should lift its head within 3 minutes post calving.*
- *Newborn calf should attain sternal recumbency within 5 minutes post calving.*
- *Newborn calf should attempt to stand within 20 minutes post calving.*
- *Newborn calf should stand spontaneously within 60-90 minutes post calving.*

Points to Remember

- Ensure calves are born in a clean, freshly bedded calving unit
- Clean nostrils and mouth which helps the calf breathe better and help prevent future breathing problems.
- Allow the mother to lick the calf clean which promotes circulation within the calf's body and prepares the calf to stand up and walk.
- Remove all the wet bedding from the cow pen and wash cow udder with clean water and dilute potassium permanganate solution.
- Cut the navel cord following proper method and dip in tincture of iodine. Dipping the navel in 7% Tr. iodine is very important in preventing navel infection.
- Colostrum should be fed early and in adequate quantity to the new born calf. A new born calf should be given 2 liters of colostrum within the first 2 hours of birth and 1-2 liters (based on size) within 12 hours of birth.
- Check the calf regularly for signs of navel ill.
- Deworm the new borne calve within 10-14 days.
- When the animal is 3 months old, contact the veterinarian for vaccination.

Newborn Calf of cows is highly susceptible to various contagious bacterial infections as well as opportunistic bacteria present in their vicinity/environment especially during early age due to immature immune system. Diarrhea, pneumonia, septicemia, endotoxemia, omphalophlebitis, osteomyelitis, meningitis, septic arthritis etc are some of the most common infections occurring in neonates. Antimicrobial therapy is considered a cornerstone of treatment for such infections in newborn calves and it is of utmost importance to start antibiotic therapy as early as possible upon anticipation of any infection. Generally broad spectrum antibiotic coverage should be started and bactericidal drugs are mostly preferred to treat neonatal infections taking into consideration the immature immune system of neonates. In cases of neonates generally large doses with longer dosage interval are administered to achieve optimum pharmacokinetic parameters to increase efficacy of antibiotic treatment.

19

Reproductive Goals for Maximum Profit in Cattle Rearing

Maintenance of optimum fertility and reproductive goals is very important for profitable and economically viable cattle rearing. It is highly desired and essential for the farmers to maintain the high reproductive efficiency in cows so that the losses incurred on infertility are reduced to the maximum extent through good managemental practices and following scientific guidelines properly.

Reproductive Traits	**Goal**
Calving interval i.e. Time between birth of one calf to another calf	365-380 days
Average days to 1st observed heat after calving	Less than 40 days
Average days open to 1st breeding after calving	50-60 days
Average days open to conception	85-100 days
Services/conception	1.5-1.7
Dry period length	45-60 days
Average age at 1st breeding of heifer*	15 months
Average age at 1st calving of heifer	24 months
% cows pregnant less than or equal to 3 AI services	90%
% cows pregnant on exam	80-85%
Abortion rate	Less than 5%
Source: Arthurs Veterinary Reproduction and Obstetrics-8th Edition